Book by

Dr. Theodore

# INTRODUCTION

It is not as difficult as you might think to maintain good health. You probably learned in school that the body has built-in mechanisms for taking care of itself. The problem is that people sometimes forget that they need to eat certain things for these built-in mechanisms to work. Every nutrient in the food they eat helps keep the body's chemistry the same, which makes it work well. Everyone should lead a healthy lifestyle. We also feel better when we take care of our physical health—we feel fitter, more relaxed, and better able to deal with things. This is even more critical when you are suffering from a mental illness. You probably can tell when you're not in your healthiest state. You might just feel "off."You might notice that you feel tired, that your digestive system isn't working as well as it should, and that you seem to get colds. Mentally, you might feel anxious or depressed and have trouble concentrating.

# Chapter 1

## INTRODUCTION

Understanding what healthy body chemistry is and how it contributes to optimal body performance and long-term health are covered in this course. You will learn about the chemicals your body makes and how these chemicals affect your body in this section. With this information, you will know which foods to include in your diet and which ones to avoid.

**What Does It Mean to Have a Balanced Body Chemistry?** The term "body chemistry" refers to all processes that occur within the body, from heartbeats to cell production. The chemicals produced by the body make it possible for all of these processes. Using this definition of body chemistry, we can say that a balanced body has the right amount of chemicals to help the body work right.

When a person's body chemistry is in balance, he or she is in good health. Your body constantly requires the nutrients provided by food to achieve and maintain this equilibrium. You get fats, vitamins, minerals, proteins (amino acids), and other nutrients that the body needs to keep running smoothly. These nutrients may cause health issues if consumed in excess or the wrong amounts.

What effects does your body chemistry have? Your biochemistry changes constantly every day. When you eat, study, work, exercise, and sleep, it changes. Sugar levels rise in the blood after eating; When you argue with someone, your blood pressure rises or your heart rate accelerates after jogging.

Your body's chemistry can either be balanced or out of balance as a result of whatever you do, so these changes can be good or bad.

When your blood pressure is normal, your weight is about right, you are neither overweight nor obese, and you have no health issues, then, your body's chemistry is in balance. On the other hand, you are more likely to have high blood pressure and other health issues if you weigh more or less than you should; then your body's chemistry is out of balance.

What is a balanced pH, and why is it important to maintain healthy body chemistry?

The amount of acid/alkaline in your body is one of the most important factors that affect balance or imbalance in your chemistry. The body's acid or alkaline content is measured in PH units. If your pH level is lower than 7, it means that your body has more acid, and if it is higher than 7, it means that your body has more alkaline. 7 is the neutral pH level.

Even though your blood's PH is slightly alkaline, medical research has shown that your body works best when your saliva and urine are slightly above 7 PH. The body can fight off fatigue and illnesses at this pH level. You can maintain your ideal weight because your metabolism functions properly.

Your body is forced to get nutrients from your vital organs to counter the acidity, which weakens your body until it is no longer able to do its job. Over time, this could lead to dangerous health problems for your body.

The following chapters will be even more helpful to you because you already know how important it is to have healthy body chemistry.

# Chapter 2
## Chemistry of the blood

When your doctor needs to find out about a possible illness, blood tests are a must. It is a part of diagnostic procedures where everyone on the healthcare team can check your actual condition to back up their physical assessment findings. Often, these blood tests are your worst enemy as they inflict pain although they are important. Understanding the blood's chemistry is the first step toward understanding the significance of these tests.

**What is Blood Chemistry?** Our body is made up of millions of chemicals that work together to make all of our organs work. They typically circulate throughout the body in the blood, where they are distributed to organ cells. Consequently, blood chemistry is defined as the actual chemical composition of our blood. Our blood chemistry changes on its own when we are ill or have ingested something harmful. Both because it needs to fight off the harmful substances (or microorganisms) and because these harmful substances have their blood chemistry that mixes with yours.

Your blood tests will also differ depending on the health condition you have. Your blood glucose changes when you eat too much sugar; A kidney problem or a damaged liver can cause your blood to turn a yellowish color and disrupt blood flow. These are just a few examples of the chemical changes that occur in our blood when we suffer an injury.

*What are the Blood Chemistry Tests?*

Depending on the symptoms that your body is exhibiting, a variety of blood tests are carried out. One type of blood test or a combination of multiple types may be ordered by your doctor. This is because our organs interact with one another in such a way that if one is damaged, the other may also be affected. Consequently, the following are typical blood tests that your doctor may order.

**Glucose test**: As a result of the growing prevalence of obesity and sedentary living, glucose testing is by far the most common blood test. Your doctor can use this to see how your body uses glucose and determine whether you have diabetes or other metabolic issues.

**SGOT and SGPT**: these two blood tests are necessary to assess your liver's condition for liver function. These two enzymes collaborate with the liver, so when the liver is damaged, they will both be released into the blood, rising. Problems with the liver are indicated by elevated SGPT and SGOT levels.

**Blood Urea Nitrogen**: A blood test called blood urea nitrogen, or BUN, is used to assess your kidney health. Your kidney filters the blood's waste, one of which is nitrogen, round-the-clock. Nitrogen enters the bloodstream unfiltered as a result of kidney damage. Therefore, kidney issues are indicated by an increase in BUN. The thyroid function tests T2 and T3, the kidney function test Creatinine, and the sodium and electrolytes test to check for dehydration are additional tests. These are the most common blood tests that your doctor may order to determine the nature of your illness and whether or not your organs are still functioning normally.

**Calcium test**: The calcium level in the blood is determined by this test. If testing shows low levels, it could mean that your parathyroid glands aren't working as hard as they should, that your diet doesn't have enough calcium, or that you don't have enough vitamin D, among other less common conditions.

High levels may indicate conditions such as overactive parathyroid glands, excessive vitamin D supplementation, kidney issues, and other concerning causes that typically necessitate additional investigation. Other parameters like albumin and total serum protein need to be tested to properly interpret calcium levels.

# Chapter 3
## The relationship between blood's biology and chemistry

Everywhere you look, you can see the connection between your biology and the chemistry of your blood. Chemicals are everywhere, and they all play a role in a variety of applications if you will observe. Additionally, our body is comprised of various chemicals that are required for proper function. This includes maintaining life, which is the focus of biology. Learn how the blood's biology and chemistry interact with one another and how they can nourish and sustain your life.

To be readable, even these letters are composed of a series of chemicals. Chemicals make up everything in your computer, from the monitor to the internal hardware. The chemical structure of everything you see serves a particular purpose. Each and everything in the world has a distinct chemical makeup if you think about it. However, the relationship between it and your blood chemistry, which is what exactly determines how your body functions, is the most crucial aspect to comprehend.

## The Relationship Defined

There are three scientific fields involved in the connection between our blood chemistry and biology: molecular biology, biochemistry, and genetics each body system rely on these to function effectively. Their definitions as well as examples

**Genetic:** The investigation of genes and ancestry. The transmission of genetic information and characteristics, such as eye color and an increased risk of a particular disease, from parents to offspring is known as heredity.

**Biochemistry**: The study of a living organism's bodily processes is known as biochemistry. Because it focuses on the specific function of molecules in the body, biochemistry is important in biology. Organ functions, the structure of cells, and the chemical components of blood are among these.

**Molecular biology**: Molecular biology, whose name comes from the word "molecule," focuses on the structure and function of cells. It entails studying a particular cell's response to specific conditions, as well as its replication and utilization of ingested substances.

The biological functions of our bodies and their connection to blood chemistry are at the heart of each of these three fields of study. The normal composition of your blood is altered when a certain chemical enters your body. This reaction occurs automatically. Depending on the chemical, this could be harmful or beneficial. Your body reacts differently to certain chemicals because of this.

**Relevance of Relationship:**
The concept of relating the body to biology and blood chemistry is regarded as entirely novel. Because of this, the practice of using it for healing and therapy is referred to as molecular medicine. Numerous biological processes, as well as physical and chemical methods, are used in molecular medicine to either identify a specific health issue or offer preventative measures. It sometimes also looks at a patient's gene expression to figure out what's causing their current condition.
The connection between biology and blood chemistry is crucial not only for maintaining daily life but also for advancing the environment. All of these chemicals have an impact on us all, either positively or negatively.

# Chapter 4
## Dangerous Chemicals to the Body

You are exposed to pollutants and chemicals that could harm your health every day. You might not be aware of the chemicals that enter your body. Therefore, even If you are in the comfort of your room, a laboratory,  hospital, hazardous chemicals may remain around you.

Despite their prevalence, you must be aware that these chemicals can only be harmful if absorbed by the body. Therefore, it is essential that you are familiar with the terms associated with chemicals before arriving at any conclusions; about whether they might be harmful or toxic. Are you aware of the distinction?

**Hazardous** – this is the term used when certain substances accumulate in a concentration that can harm your body.

**Toxic:** When a substance has caused harm to the body, especially when it reaches a certain level, it is referred to as toxic.

## The Pathways Spelled Out

Therefore, the term "toxic" simply refers to the fact that a chemical can have negative effects at a given concentration. Scientists and other professionals typically use percentages to define toxicity and measure it in terms of the amount that can kill.

Typically, tests are conducted on rats. Since a chemical is considered toxic if it causes 50% of deaths, these rats perform a heroic task in defining toxicity. Hazardous chemicals, on the other hand, may or may not be toxic, so they should be handled with care to avoid danger.

Now that you know the difference between chemicals that are harmful and toxic, the next thing you need to know is how they typically enter the body. Our bodies may absorb these harmful chemicals without our knowledge. We occasionally inhale them; They are absorbed even through our skin and ingested. They invade in a way that makes it impossible for them to get into our system.

When we consume: You can only actually allow these chemicals to enter your body through your mouth. A potential risk is eating in a contaminated area or drinking unclean water or food.

Upon inhalation: Chemical intrusion is more likely to affect those who work in hazardous conditions. These chemicals enter your body by first entering your lungs and then contacting your body's blood vessels. They begin their journey into the system via these vessels.

When we take in: A series of cells that are capable of absorbing substances make up your skin, eyes included. This is how your lotions and topical medications absorb their chemicals. As a result, a harmful chemical that enters your skin will find its way through your skin.

You need to know these things about the chemicals and pollution that could get into your system. A material's health effects can still be used to describe its danger. Mutagens alter the DNA of cells and cause cancer, irritants aggravate our body tissues, and narcotics are depressants. In addition, sensitizers cause allergies, teratogens affect pregnant women's fetuses, and poisons cause internal damage. Visit your doctor right away for additional information.

# Chapter 5

## Good chemical for the body

A person needs to exercise to maintain their health and fitness. It would have physiological advantages as well as physical advantages for your body.

The body produces beneficial chemicals while exercising. Running, for instance, is an exercise that starts a chain reaction in your body that causes chemicals called neurotransmitters to be activated in a brain cycle.

While running, neurotransmitters can release feelings of happiness and excitement, as well as feelings of exhaustion after exercise.

**Endorphins:** When you feel pain or stress, your body releases chemicals called endorphins (hormones). They are released while having fun doing things like exercise, getting a massage, eating, and having sex. Endorphins aid in pain relief, stress reduction, and improved well-being.

The limbic and prefrontal regions of a person's brain are the targets of endorphins. Emotions and feelings are controlled by these parts of the brain. The runner's high level of activity is related to the release of endorphins. This chemical has the potential to alleviate pain and improve the runner's mood.

A German researcher's study found that people who run every day are more tolerant than those who don't. Addiction is also linked to this chemical. Endorphins are thought to be released by drug users, which leads to an addiction to using drugs. The same applies to runners; they would describe it as "addictive."

**Serotonin:** A person's mood, appetite, sleep cycle, and libido are all controlled by the chemical serotonin. It is also released when you eat turkey and carbohydrates, in addition to when you exercise. Artificial serotonin is a medication used to alleviate depression symptoms and improve mood in some cases of depression. Even after you exercise, the effects of serotonin last longer in your body, making you feel better overall.

**Neurotrophic Factor**: A neurotransmitter that helps the brain, specifically the hippocampus, is neurotrophic. The brain's overall health and improvement in memory are both attributed to this chemical. Experts say that people with depression don't have enough of this neurotransmitter.

It is possible to increase mental alertness and happiness through exercise. However, during an exercise session, the body only releases a certain amount of this neurotransmitter. The amount of neurotransmitter released will not increase even if you exercise longer.

A person who exercises regularly is more likely to feel happy and eat well. This is because the body releases "feel-good" neurotransmitters, which help a person stay fit and healthy mentally as well as physically. A person's happiness will be maintained and their risk of developing depression will decrease as these beneficial chemicals are released.

These neurotransmitters will also keep things in balance when a person experiences a feeling. Therefore, if you want to maintain physical and mental health and happiness, you should exercise regularly. Unless you regularly exercise your body, these chemicals won't get into your body. Including exercise in your week's schedule will not only help you get ready for work, but it will also help you feel less stressed.

# Chapter 6
## The Effects of the Chemicals' Chemistry

Chemicals and health are easy to connect to. You've probably heard of organic chemicals or organic compounds, which are generally defined as substances made up of molecules with carbon atoms. And what's more? All living things contain these compounds, which are the basis for all biological and natural processes.

**Learn about chemicals that can either help or hurt you with healthy chemistry for optimal health.**

**Why the Chemical Aversion?** Chemicals play a significant role in our ability to function as living things. However, in recent times, people have been experiencing negative emotions at the mere mention of the word chemical. Chemical warfare is mentioned, and people are seen stumbling around, gasping for air. When someone who cares about their health hears that vegetables are grown with chemical or synthetic fertilizers, they shudder at the thought of eating such foods.

With chemicals, scientists can accomplish a lot. They are capable of combining a variety of chemicals to produce life- or health-saving solutions as well as terrifying weapons, such as the chemical weapons we frequently hear about.

**Benefits for the Health Industry:** Without knowledge of how chemicals work in the body, the health industry would not be what it is today. They wouldn't know how to use the PH measurement, which tells how acidic or alkaline the body is, and they wouldn't know how to make programs to fix health issues. Worse yet, they wouldn't be aware of any preventative measures.

**Chemistry of chemical:** A chemical affects another chemical. This is the chemistry of chemicals. This knowledge is very important to the health industry because the impact or reaction falls under the realm of chemistry. How should acidity, which is associated with numerous health issues, be mitigated? A health professional, on the other hand, will advise avoiding tea, milk, banana, cucumber, melon, spicy chutneys, pickles, and vinegar. Even if he knew about chemicals and chemistry, he couldn't have told the patient what to avoid or what to take.

Knowing what chemicals do for and to the body as well as what will happen if two chemicals with different properties are combined is, therefore, the key to maintaining good health and developing treatments.

The healthcare industry is one of the primary beneficiaries of the significant advancements that the field of chemistry has made over the years. Because of this, the industry hasn't changed much, and now and then, new health plans and products based on new information appear on the market. The industry's best products, on the other hand, are those that simply balance the body's chemical levels to support and preserve the body's natural and correct biological processes.

Does this imply that all available health products are efficient? Well, people have options. Specifications—nutrition facts for health products or chemical content for non-food solutions—must be considered. The state of the body should also be taken into account when making the decision, as the chemicals that are absorbed by the products can cause adverse reactions in the body.

# Chapter 7

## Reasons Why You Should Avoid the Bad Chemicals

If not handled with care, chemicals, especially those you use to clean your home, can be dangerous. Some industrial cleaners' marketing strategies have been successful in raising public awareness of the significance of cleanliness. However, they also failed to provide adequate warnings about the potential health risks posed by these chemicals. Here are some good reasons not to use harmful chemicals so that you can choose safer options.

## Reason

1. **The Effect of Triclosan**: This synthetic is utilized normally in cleansers that are made to be against bacteria. While these potent chemicals may kill bacteria

in your body, they also pose risks. Because they interact with your thyroid glands, they affect your metabolism. When it reacts with contaminated water, this can also pose a threat to aquatic animals. Avoid using this product too much. It has the potential to be harmful and will make your body more resistant to other antibiotics.

2. **The warning about Ammonia**: When used in household cleaners, ammonia can be inhaled. This chemical could harm children's health if they inhale it. Try cleaning your sink or tiles with baking soda as an alternative. They are safe and natural to use.

3. .**The Dangers of Pesticides**: Even if marketing campaigns portray pesticides as "natural," you are pretty sure that they are poison. These chemicals kill the soil, preventing the plant from receiving nutrients.

4. **The Drawbacks of Grilling**: Grilling causes your food to slightly char, which results in the production of heterocyclic amines. Since this substance is cancer-causing, remove it from your plate.

5. .**Precautions for Sunless Tanning**: Even if you stay away from the sun's harmful rays, sunless tanning still contains potent chemicals that have the potential to irritate the skin and cause other skin problems.

6: **Dangers of Smoke Belching**: You are aware of the carbon monoxide damage caused by smoke to your lungs. You can now begin cleaning your car and make your surroundings much cleaner.

7. **Nail Polish Alert**: it contains butyl acetate, an active ingredient that can be harmful to breathe in, especially if you are around children. Make sure to use it in an open area or away from kids.

# Chapter 8

## Reasons Why You Should Only Have the Good Chemicals

You are provided with information about the dangers that chemicals pose to your body from the chapter that came before it. Not all of them are bad. Some chemicals are labeled as safe and effective. You should choose safe chemicals for these reasons, as well as what to do if you can't avoid them.

## Substitution or Elimination Process

Either replacing harmful chemicals with safer alternatives or completely avoiding their use is the most common method for reducing their risk. The following are good alternatives to harmful chemicals:

❖ water-based Paints can be used in place

of those that are water-based.

- ❖ Getting rid of grease by using trichloromethane instead of trichloroethylene

You can also eliminate the products from your surroundings. For instance, hair sprays and antibacterial soaps should be completely avoided. The most important thing to keep in mind here is to stop using harmful chemicals altogether or to buy less harmful chemicals.

**Protecting Yourself from Danger:** The majority of our lives are spent in danger. We still come into contact with these chemicals every day at work. As a result, you need to strengthen your immune system to protect yourself from danger. Although our body is capable of defending itself against invasion, our compromised immune system puts us at risk for infection.

Vitamin supplements are necessary for a stronger immune system, so if you eat poorly, take them. It is preferable to wear a mask and laboratory gown if you are frequently exposed to chemicals. Because it can carry contaminants when touched or inhaled, equipment should sometimes be moved to a location where public exposure is minimal.

**The Crucial Role of Proper Airflow:** To guard against harmful chemicals, it is working in an environment that allows air circulation is critical airborne chemicals can enter a room and invade the entire space, particularly if there is only a limited exit. As a result, fresh oxygen will continue to fill the space as long as there is adequate ventilation, so these harmful chemicals will not remain for an extended period. The chemicals will be less likely to pose a threat as a result of this.

**The Advantages of Proper Hygiene:** Above all else, it's best to start with yourself before cleaning your surroundings and ensuring that safer chemicals are used. Make sure your body is clean before going to work or going to bed to practice good hygiene. If you work in an environment where you are constantly exposed to chemicals, this is especially important. These harmful chemicals can adhere to your clothing and skin, putting your health and the health of those around you in danger.

If you have to use a certain chemical, you need to use safe chemicals and take some safety precautions for these reasons. Since chemicals are all around you, you should always take the necessary precautions and protect yourself.

# Chapter 9
## Things to think about when choosing which chemicals to put in your body

The lining of your cells, which can be found in your lungs, skin, or mouth, is where the majority of the body's foreign substances typically enter the system. After that, it enters your body's fluids, of which there are two types: intracellular and interstitial.

Fluids make up almost 60% of your body weight and make up your entire body. These harmful chemicals can enter your body fluids and invade one or more organs.

Because of this, you need to choose the right product with more care to avoid ingesting harmful chemicals. When choosing the chemicals that our bodies absorb, the following considerations need to be made.

# Discover how chemicals can enter the body.

Since these were briefly discussed in the preceding chapter, we now move on to the specifics. Your interstitial fluid—the fluid that surrounds your cells—can be contaminated with a chemical. Unlike your blood, which continuously circulates inside and around your heart to keep it clean, these fluids are not blood. Instead, it stays in one place, where nutrients and water flow in and out. Therefore, if a harmful chemical is present in your interstitial fluid, it will not be carried by your blood and will instead remain in one part of your body, resulting in infections.

Before the chemical can completely enter a cell, it must first penetrate the cell's membrane. It must first enter the blood vessels before eventually entering the organ it wishes to invade. The chemicals' ability may differ depending on their molecular structure, solubility, polarity, and other characteristics. Additionally, this explains why a particular chemical causes distinct health issues from others.

**Be aware of the exposure route:** This specifies whether or not a particular chemical will inevitably be eliminated. Some are absorbed into the bloodstream and eliminated further. For instance, a particular chemical targets your liver first when it invades your body. We are all aware that the liver is an important filter that can eliminate hazardous chemicals.

As a result, a specific chemical will be going through a process called "downstream," during which it will be eliminated or destroyed. This also explains why certain medications are given in different ways depending on how they work. Some medications should not pass through the liver to reach organs, while others must target the organ itself.

They are stored in the body Frequently, the chemicals may enter the body and become entangled in plasma proteins. Plasma proteins are storage cells that can put the chemical into dormancy. This is because the plasma's proteins prevent the toxins from harming anything. That results in the rapid binding of a particular chemical to a protein.

When deciding which chemicals to put in your body, these are the things to keep in mind. Some of them invade, while others are destroyed. Check your product out at your neighborhood stores to learn everything you can about it.

# CONCLUDING
## Chemical and optimal health

Many of the materials we use in our environment can be harmful to our health. Through direct body contact, ingestion, or internal absorption, these chemicals affect our health. We must know the distinction between "hazardous" and "toxic" chemicals to comprehend the significance of chemicals to optimal health and evaluate their potential health effects.

**Hazard:** A concentration's potential danger or risk to the body is referred to as a "hazard."A material's toxicity is an inherent property, whereas a substance's hazard is its probability of occurring. Consider that even if a material is extremely toxic, it may still be non-hazardous when handled appropriately to better comprehend this. On the other hand, some substances, like acid in an open container, may be less harmful but pose a significant risk due to their prevalence and packaging.

**Toxicity**: The degree to which a substance or chemical can harm any organism after coming into contact with a specific part of the body is known as toxicity. The material is toxic if it causes unintended effects. The process is as follows: A material's level of toxicity is proportional to the amount of time it takes to become ingested, absorbed, or in contact with another substance. To cause more harm to the body, a greater quantity is required if the substance is less toxic. To determine the level of toxicity, these chemicals are tested on animals, typically rats.

## Various Entryways:

Toxic substances can enter a person's body in three different ways. Such are:

• Through oral ingestion, which refers to the toxic substance being swallowed by the mouth;

• Through skin or eye absorption, which refers to the material or substance coming into direct contact with the skin and being absorbed through the pores in the skin or eyes;

• Through nasal or oral inhalation, which refers to the

process by which a chemical substance is inhaled through the air in the environment through the nose or mouth.

## Classification of chemical substance

Numerous chemicals have the potential to harm the body. It is crucial to know which substances can be harmful and how they will affect the body. The harmful substances that fall under this category, along with some good examples, are as follows:

• Irritants that can irritate the tissues when they come into contact, like ammonia and nitrogen dioxide

• Narcotics or anesthetics that can harm the central nervous system, like chloroform and xylene

• System poisons, like carbon tetrachloride and halogenated hydrocarbons, that can hurt internal organs

• Carcinogens, like arsenic, benzene, inorganic chromium salts, beryllium

• Teratogens, such as thalidomide and possibly steroids, are harmful to pregnant women because they have the potential to cause defects in the fetus

• Sensitizer agents, such as cutting oils, isocyanates in polyurethane foam operations, paint spraying operations, and some laboratory solvents, have the potential to cause allergic reactions.

Our environment contains numerous chemical substances that can be harmful to our health. To avoid potentially fatal effects on our bodies, we must be aware of their effects and use them
appropriately. Both optimal health and awareness
of chemicals are very important.
While there are numerous harmful and toxic chemicals all around us, there are also beneficial chemicals that we require for survival. We need to use these chemicals in moderation for optimal. health. Before putting any chemicals in our bodies, it is highly recommended that we learn more about them and what they can do for us. Both the world as a whole and our bodies are huge balls of chemicals and other substances. We can live our best lives if we know how we interact with one another.